Women Over 50 Intermittent Fasting Cookbook

Michele Nora

Disclaimer

Please bear in mind that the information in this book is strictly educational. The data presented here is claimed to be credible and trustworthy. The author provides no implied or explicit assurance of accuracy for specific
individual instances.
It is important that you consult with a skilled practitioner, such as your doctor, before initiating any diet or lifestyle changes. The information in this book should not be used in place of expert advice or professional assistance.
The author, publisher, and distributor fully disclaim any and all liability, loss, damage, or risk suffered by anybody who relies on the information in this book, whether directly or indirectly.
All intellectual property rights are intact. The content in this book should not be copied in any way, mechanically, electronically, by photocopying, or by any other means available.

CONTENTS

Introduction

Welcome to the transformative journey towards a healthier, more vibrant you. In the vast realm of health and wellness, the decision to prioritize your well-being is a powerful and empowering choice, especially for women over 50. This introduction serves as an invitation to explore the world of intermittent fasting, a lifestyle approach that can play a pivotal role in achieving and sustaining optimal health at this stage of life.

Before embarking on this journey together, I want to express my deepest gratitude to all those who have contributed to the creation of this cookbook. From the researchers and scientists whose work has illuminated the benefits of intermittent fasting for women over 50, to the culinary experts and nutritionists who have crafted the delicious recipes within these pages, this collaborative effort reflects a shared commitment to empowering women to live their healthiest lives.

Allow me to introduce myself. As the author of this cookbook, my journey into the world of health and wellness has been driven by a passion for empowering individuals to make informed choices about their well-being. With a background in nutrition and a deep understanding of the unique needs of women over 50, I have endeavored to create a resource that not only educates but also inspires positive change. This cookbook is a culmination of my dedication to helping you navigate the path to a healthier, more fulfilling life.

As we age, our bodies undergo various changes, and the importance of mindful nutrition becomes increasingly evident. Intermittent fasting emerges as a powerful tool tailored to the specific needs of women over 50. In this section, we delve into the scientific foundations of intermittent fasting, exploring how it addresses age-related challenges, enhances metabolic health, and promotes overall well-being. From hormonal balance to cognitive function, discover why intermittent fasting is not just a trend but a transformative approach to aging gracefully.

Navigating a new lifestyle can be overwhelming, but fear not. This section provides a roadmap for effectively utilizing the resources within this cookbook. From understanding the basics of intermittent fasting to making informed choices about nutrition, each chapter is designed to build upon the last. Whether you are a beginner seeking a comprehensive introduction or an experienced fast learner looking for new recipes and insights, the organization of this cookbook ensures that you can tailor your experience to meet your unique needs. Take a moment to familiarize yourself with the structure, and feel free to customize your journey toward a healthier you.

Chapter 1: Understanding Intermittent Fasting

Intermittent fasting (IF) has gained significant attention in recent years as a potential strategy for improving health and well-being. This chapter delves into the science behind intermittent fasting, explores its benefits for women over 50, and dispels common myths and misconceptions surrounding this dietary approach.

The Science Behind Intermittent Fasting

Intermittent fasting is not a new concept; it has historical roots in various cultures and religions. However, its recent resurgence is fueled by a growing body of scientific research supporting its potential health benefits. At its core, intermittent fasting involves cycling between periods of eating and fasting. The most common methods include the 16/8 method (16 hours of fasting with an 8-hour eating window), the 5:2 method (normal eating for five days and restricted caloric intake for two non-consecutive days), and the eat-stop-eat method (24-hour fasts once or twice a week).

The science behind intermittent fasting is multifaceted. During the fasting period, the body undergoes metabolic changes, including a decrease in insulin levels and an increase in norepinephrine, promoting fat breakdown for energy. Additionally, cellular repair processes, such as autophagy, are activated, leading to the removal of damaged cells and cellular components. These mechanisms contribute to improved insulin sensitivity, weight management, and overall cellular health.

Benefits for Women Over 50

Women over 50 experience unique physiological changes, including hormonal fluctuations and a gradual decline in metabolic rate. Intermittent fasting offers several potential benefits for this demographic. One key advantage is its positive impact on insulin sensitivity, which becomes increasingly important as individuals age. Improved insulin sensitivity can help manage blood sugar levels and reduce the risk of type 2 diabetes.

Furthermore, intermittent fasting may support cardiovascular health by reducing risk factors such as high blood pressure and cholesterol levels. The potential for weight management is crucial for women in this age group, as maintaining a healthy weight is associated with a lower risk of chronic diseases and improved overall well-being. Cognitively, intermittent fasting has been linked to enhanced brain health and a reduced risk of neurodegenerative diseases. This is particularly relevant for women over 50 who may be concerned about cognitive decline associated with aging.

Common Myths and Misconceptions:

Despite its growing popularity, intermittent fasting is not without its share of myths and misconceptions. One common misconception is that it leads to muscle loss. However, when practiced correctly with an adequate intake of protein, intermittent fasting can preserve muscle mass and even promote its growth.

Another myth is that intermittent fasting is only effective for weight loss. While it can be a powerful tool for weight management, intermittent fasting also offers a range of health benefits beyond shedding pounds. These include improved metabolic health, better blood sugar control, and enhanced cellular repair mechanisms.

Additionally, there's a misconception that intermittent fasting is not suitable for women. In reality, many women, including those over 50, have successfully incorporated intermittent fasting into their lifestyles. It's essential, however, for women to tailor their approach to accommodate their unique hormonal fluctuations and nutritional needs.

In conclusion, understanding the science behind intermittent fasting is crucial for harnessing its benefits. For women over 50, this dietary approach can offer a range of advantages, from improved metabolic health to cognitive well-being. By dispelling common myths and misconceptions, individuals can make informed decisions about whether intermittent fasting aligns with their health and lifestyle goals.

Chapter 2: Getting Started with Intermittent Fasting

Embarking on an intermittent fasting journey requires thoughtful consideration and planning. This chapter focuses on the initial steps of getting started with intermittent fasting, covering the assessment of readiness, choosing the right fasting method, and establishing realistic goals.

Assessing Your Readiness

Before diving into intermittent fasting, it's crucial to assess your readiness and determine if this dietary approach aligns with your lifestyle, health status, and personal preferences. Consider factors such as your current eating habits, medical conditions, and daily routine. Individuals with certain medical conditions or those who are pregnant should consult with a healthcare professional before starting intermittent fasting.

Readiness also involves a mental and emotional assessment. Intermittent fasting can be a significant shift in eating patterns, and being mentally prepared for this change is essential. Reflect on your willingness to embrace a new approach to eating and whether you have the support and resources needed for a successful transition.

Choosing the Right Fasting Method

There are various intermittent fasting methods, and selecting the one that fits your lifestyle and goals is pivotal. The 16/8 method, which involves a daily 16-hour fasting window and an 8-hour eating window, is popular and adaptable. The 5:2 method, where you eat normally for five days and restrict caloric intake for two non-consecutive days, offers flexibility. The eat-stop-eat method involves 24-hour fasts once or twice a week.

Consider your daily schedule, work commitments, and social activities when choosing a fasting method. The method should seamlessly integrate into your routine to enhance sustainability. Additionally, take into account individual preferences regarding meal timing and frequency.

Establishing Realistic Goals

Setting realistic and achievable goals is fundamental to a successful intermittent fasting journey. Goals can vary, from weight management and improved metabolic health to enhanced mental clarity and energy levels. Begin by identifying your primary objectives and breaking them down into smaller, manageable steps.

Realistic goals are specific, measurable, achievable, relevant, and time-bound (SMART). For instance, if weight loss is a goal, specify the amount of weight you aim to lose within a realistic timeframe. Regularly assess and adjust your goals based on your progress and evolving priorities.
It's essential to acknowledge that intermittent fasting is not a one-size-fits-all solution. Goals should be personalized to align with your individual needs and health aspirations. Be patient with the process, as it may take time to adapt to the new eating pattern and observe tangible results.

In conclusion, getting started with intermittent fasting involves a thoughtful assessment of readiness, the selection of an appropriate fasting method, and the establishment of realistic goals. By approaching intermittent fasting with a well-informed and personalized strategy, individuals can enhance the likelihood of long-term success and enjoy the numerous potential health benefits associated with this dietary approach.

Chapter 3: Exercise and Movement for Women Over 50

As women transition into their 50s, maintaining a healthy and active lifestyle becomes increasingly crucial for overall well-being. This chapter delves into the importance of exercise and movement for women over 50, emphasizing the need for tailored workouts, the role of strength training and cardio, and the incorporation of mind-body practices for holistic health.

Tailoring Workouts to Your Body

Women over 50 often experience changes in muscle mass, bone density, and hormonal balance. Therefore, it's essential to tailor workouts to accommodate these physiological shifts. Focus on exercises that enhance flexibility, balance, and joint mobility to counteract the effects of aging. Low-impact activities, such as swimming, walking, or yoga, can be particularly beneficial for maintaining joint health.

Consider individual fitness levels and any pre-existing health conditions when designing a workout routine. Customizing workouts to address specific needs and preferences ensures that exercise remains enjoyable, sustainable, and minimizes the risk of injury.

The Role of Strength Training and Cardio

Incorporating both strength training and cardiovascular exercise is pivotal for women over 50. Strength training helps counteract the natural decline in muscle mass and bone density, reducing the risk of osteoporosis. Weight-bearing exercises, such as lifting weights or bodyweight exercises, can promote bone health.

Cardiovascular exercise, on the other hand, supports heart health, boosts metabolism, and contributes to weight management. Activities like brisk walking, cycling, or dancing can be effective and enjoyable forms of cardiovascular exercise. Striking a balance between strength training and cardio ensures a comprehensive approach to fitness.

Embracing Mind-Body Practices for Holistic Health

Holistic health involves nurturing the connection between the mind and body. Mind-body practices, such as yoga, tai chi, and meditation, play a crucial role in promoting overall well-being for women over 50. These practices offer a range of benefits, including stress reduction, improved mental clarity, and enhanced emotional resilience.

Yoga, in particular, combines physical postures, breath control, and meditation, providing a holistic approach to fitness. Tai chi, with its slow and flowing movements, improves balance and flexibility while calming the mind. Incorporating these practices into a fitness routine fosters a sense of mindfulness and contributes to a more balanced and centered lifestyle.

14-Day Intermittent Fasting Meal Plan

Day 1:
- **Breakfast:** Greek Yogurt Parfait with Granola and Berries (Page 22)
- **Lunch:** Quinoa and Black Bean Salad (Page 32)
- **Dinner:** Baked Salmon with Lemon and Dill (Page 47)
- **Snack:** Hummus and Veggie Sticks (Page 62)

Day 2:
- **Breakfast:** Blueberry Almond Chia Pudding (Page 19)
- **Lunch:** Grilled Chicken Caesar Wrap (Page 33)
- **Dinner:** Teriyaki Turkey Lettuce Wraps (Page 52)
- **Snack:** Almond and Coconut Energy Bites (Page 62)

Day 3:
- **Breakfast:** Apple Cinnamon Overnight Oats (Page 27)
- **Lunch:** Lentil and Vegetable Soup (Page 34)
- **Dinner:** Stir-Fried Tofu with Broccoli and Sesame Seeds (Page 57)
- **Snack:** Cottage Cheese with Pineapple Chunks (Page 66)

Day 4:
- **Breakfast:** Quinoa Porridge with Mixed Berries (Page 20)
- **Lunch:** Greek Salad with Grilled Shrimp (Page 35)
- **Dinner:** Butternut Squash and Sage Risotto (Page 53)
- **Snack:** Mixed Nuts and Dried Fruit Trail Mix (Page 67)

Day 5:
- **Breakfast:** Sweet Potato Hash with Poached Eggs (Page 23)
- **Lunch:** Zucchini Noodles with Pesto and Cherry Tomatoes (Page 36)
- **Dinner:** Cilantro Lime Grilled Chicken (Page 54)
- **Snack:** Avocado and Tomato Salsa (Page 67)

Day 6:
- **Breakfast:** Banana Nut Smoothie Bowl (Page 25)
- **Lunch:** Caprese Salad with Balsamic Glaze (Page 39)
- **Dinner:** Spinach and Mushroom Quiche (Page 59)
- **Snack:** Roasted Chickpeas with Cumin and Paprika (Page 68)

Day 7:
- **Breakfast:** Veggie and Cheese Frittata (Page 29)
- **Lunch:** Asian-Inspired Chicken Salad (Page 39)
- **Dinner:** Quinoa Stuffed Bell Peppers with Black Beans (Page 55)
- **Snack:** Hard-Boiled Eggs with Paprika (Page 65)

Day 8:
- **Breakfast:** Turmeric and Ginger Infused Smoothie (Page 30)
- **Lunch:** Sweet Potato and Kale Salad with Tahini Dressing (Page 40)
- **Dinner:** Mediterranean Chickpea Salad (Page 61)
- **Snack:** Apple Slices with Almond Butter (Page 65)

Day 9:
- **Breakfast:** Cottage Cheese and Pineapple Bowl (Page 24)
- **Lunch:** Broccoli and Cheddar Stuffed Chicken Breast (Page 41)
- **Dinner:** Spinach and Feta Omelette (Page 21)
- **Snack:** Edamame with Sea Salt (Page 63)

Day 10:

- **Breakfast:** Almond Butter Toast with Sliced Strawberries (Page 29)
- **Lunch:** Tuna Salad Lettuce Cups (Page 42)
- **Dinner:** Baked Cod with Mediterranean Salsa (Page 56)
- **Snack:** Greek Yogurt with Honey and Walnuts (Page 64)

Day 11:

- **Breakfast:** Quinoa Bowl with Roasted Vegetables and Tofu (Page 43)
- **Lunch:** Eggplant and Tomato Stack with Mozzarella (Page 44)
- **Dinner:** Grilled Vegetable and Goat Cheese Quesadillas (Page 58)
- **Snack:** Mixed Nuts and Dried Fruit Trail Mix (Page 67)

Day 12:

- **Breakfast:** Blueberry Almond Butter Smoothie (Page 86)
- **Lunch:** Turkey and Avocado Lettuce Wraps (Page 37)
- **Dinner:** Pistachio and Cranberry Bark (Page 79)
- **Snack:** Chia Seed Pudding with Mango (Page 73)

Day 13:

- **Breakfast:** Mango Turmeric Smoothie (Page 82)
- **Lunch:** Cauliflower Fried Rice (Page 45)
- **Dinner:** Stir-Fried Tofu with Broccoli and Sesame Seeds (Page 57)
- **Snack:** Raspberry Almond Bliss Balls (Page 74)

Day 14:

- **Breakfast:** Strawberry Kiwi Smoothie with Chia Seeds (Page 89)
- **Lunch:** Chickpea and Spinach Stuffed Bell Peppers (Page 38)
- **Dinner:** Teriyaki Turkey Lettuce Wraps (Page 52)
- **Snack:** Hummus and Veggie Sticks (Page 62)

Breakfast

Avocado and Egg Breakfast Wrap

- *Total Time:* 15 minutes
- *Servings:* 2

Ingredients:

- 2 large whole wheat or spinach tortillas
- 1 ripe avocado, sliced
- 4 large eggs
- Salt and pepper to taste
- 1 tablespoon olive oil
- 1/2 cup cherry tomatoes, halved
- 1/4 cup feta cheese, crumbled
- Fresh cilantro, chopped (for garnish, optional)

Directions:

1. In a non-stick skillet, heat olive oil over medium heat.
2. Crack the eggs into the skillet, season with salt and pepper, and scramble until fully cooked.
3. Warm the tortillas in a separate pan or microwave.
4. Assemble the wraps: Place sliced avocado on each tortilla, add scrambled eggs, halved cherry tomatoes, and crumbled feta.
5. Garnish with fresh cilantro if desired.
6. Fold the sides of the tortilla over the filling to create a wrap.

Nutritional Information (per serving):

- Calories: 380
- Protein: 16g
- Fat: 26g
- Carbohydrates: 27g
- Fiber: 8g

Blueberry Almond Chia Pudding

- *Total Time:* 4 hours (including chilling time)
- *Servings:* 4

Ingredients:
- 1 cup almond milk
- 1/4 cup chia seeds
- 1 tablespoon maple syrup
- 1/2 teaspoon almond extract
- 1/2 cup fresh blueberries
- 2 tablespoons sliced almonds (for topping)

Directions:
1. In a bowl, whisk together almond milk, chia seeds, maple syrup, and almond extract.
2. Let the mixture sit for 10 minutes, then whisk again to prevent clumps.
3. Cover and refrigerate for at least 4 hours or overnight.
4. Before serving, stir the chia pudding and layer it with fresh blueberries and sliced almonds.

Nutritional Information (per serving):
- Calories: 120
- Protein: 3g
- Fat: 7g
- Carbohydrates: 13g
- Fiber: 7g

Quinoa Porridge with Mixed Berries

- *Total Time:* 20 minutes
- *Servings:* 2

Ingredients:
- 1/2 cup quinoa, rinsed
- 1 cup almond milk
- 1 tablespoon honey
- 1/2 teaspoon vanilla extract
- 1/2 cup mixed berries (strawberries, blueberries, raspberries)
- 2 tablespoons chopped nuts (e.g., almonds or walnuts)

Directions:
1. In a saucepan, combine quinoa, almond milk, honey, and vanilla extract.
2. Bring to a boil, then reduce heat and simmer until quinoa is cooked and mixture thickens (about 15 minutes).
3. Stir in mixed berries.
4. Serve the quinoa porridge topped with chopped nuts.

Nutritional Information (per serving):
- Calories: 280
- Protein: 7g
- Fat: 6g
- Carbohydrates: 49g
- Fiber: 6g

Smoked Salmon and Cream Cheese Bagel

- *Total Time:* 10 minutes
- *Servings:* 2

Ingredients:

- 2 whole-grain bagels, sliced and toasted
- 4 oz smoked salmon
- 1/2 cup cream cheese
- 1 tablespoon capers
- Red onion, thinly sliced
- Fresh dill (for garnish)

Directions:

1. Spread cream cheese on the toasted bagel halves.
2. Layer smoked salmon on top of the cream cheese.
3. Scatter capers and red onion slices over the salmon.
4. Garnish with fresh dill.

Nutritional Information (per serving):

- Calories: 340
- Protein: 20g
- Fat: 15g
- Carbohydrates: 30g
- Fiber: 3g

Spinach and Feta Omelette

- *Total Time:* 15 minutes
- *Servings:* 1

Ingredients:

- 2 large eggs
- Salt and pepper to taste

- 1/2 cup fresh spinach, chopped
- 2 tablespoons feta cheese, crumbled
- 1/4 cup cherry tomatoes, halved
- 1 teaspoon olive oil

Directions:
1. In a bowl, whisk together eggs, salt, and pepper.
2. Heat olive oil in a non-stick skillet over medium heat.
3. Add chopped spinach and cook until wilted.
4. Pour the whisked eggs over the spinach, swirling to ensure even distribution.
5. Sprinkle crumbled feta and halved cherry tomatoes over one half of the omelette.
6. Once the eggs are set, fold the omelette in half and slide it onto a plate.

Nutritional Information:
- Calories: 320
- Protein: 20g
- Fat: 24g
- Carbohydrates: 5g
- Fiber: 2g

Greek Yogurt Parfait with Granola and Berries

- *Total Time:* 10 minutes
- *Servings:* 2

Ingredients:
- 1 cup Greek yogurt
- 1 cup granola
- 1 cup mixed berries (strawberries, blueberries, raspberries)

- Honey for drizzling
- Mint leaves for garnish (optional)

Directions:
1. In serving glasses or bowls, layer Greek yogurt, granola, and mixed berries.
2. Repeat the layers until the glass is filled.
3. Drizzle honey over the top.
4. Garnish with mint leaves if desired.

Nutritional Information (per serving):
- Calories: 350
- Protein: 15g
- Fat: 10g
- Carbohydrates: 50g
- Fiber: 8g

Sweet Potato Hash with Poached Eggs

- *Total Time:* 25 minutes
- *Servings:* 2

Ingredients:
- 2 medium sweet potatoes, peeled and grated
- 1 onion, finely chopped
- 2 tablespoons olive oil
- Salt and pepper to taste
- 4 large eggs
- Fresh parsley for garnish

Directions:
1. Heat olive oil in a skillet over medium heat.
2. Add chopped onions and cook until softened.

3. Add grated sweet potatoes to the skillet, season with salt and pepper, and cook until golden brown.
4. Meanwhile, poach the eggs in simmering water.
5. Serve the sweet potato hash topped with poached eggs.
6. Garnish with fresh parsley.

Nutritional Information (per serving):
- Calories: 320
- Protein: 12g
- Fat: 15g
- Carbohydrates: 40g
- Fiber: 6g

Cottage Cheese and Pineapple Bowl

- *Total Time:* 5 minutes
- *Servings:* 1

Ingredients:
- 1 cup cottage cheese
- 1/2 cup fresh pineapple chunks
- 2 tablespoons chopped nuts (e.g., almonds or walnuts)
- Drizzle of honey (optional)

Directions:
1. In a bowl, combine cottage cheese and fresh pineapple chunks.
2. Sprinkle chopped nuts over the top.
3. Drizzle with honey if desired.

Nutritional Information (per serving):
- Calories: 250

- Protein: 25g
- Fat: 10g
- Carbohydrates: 15g
- Fiber: 2g

Banana Nut Smoothie Bowl

- *Total Time:* 5 minutes
- *Servings:* 1

Ingredients:

- 1 ripe banana, frozen
- 1/2 cup Greek yogurt
- 1/4 cup almond milk
- 1 tablespoon almond butter
- Handful of granola
- Sliced banana and chopped nuts for topping

Directions:

1. In a blender, combine frozen banana, Greek yogurt, almond milk, and almond butter.
2. Blend until smooth and creamy.
3. Pour the smoothie into a bowl.
4. Top with granola, sliced banana, and chopped nuts.

Nutritional Information (per serving):

- Calories: 380
- Protein: 15g
- Fat: 18g
- Carbohydrates: 45g
- Fiber: 7g

Whole Grain Pancakes with Maple Syrup

- *Total Time:* 20 minutes
- *Servings:* 2

Ingredients:

- 1 cup whole wheat flour
- 1 tablespoon baking powder
- 1 tablespoon sugar
- 1 egg
- 1 cup milk
- 1 tablespoon melted butter
- Maple syrup for drizzling

Directions:

1. In a bowl, whisk together whole wheat flour, baking powder, and sugar.
2. In a separate bowl, beat the egg and mix in milk and melted butter.
3. Combine wet and dry ingredients, stirring until just combined.
4. Heat a griddle or non-stick pan over medium heat.
5. Pour 1/4 cup batter for each pancake onto the griddle.
6. Cook until bubbles form on the surface, then flip and cook until golden brown.
7. Drizzle with maple syrup before serving.

Nutritional Information (per serving):

- Calories: 320
- Protein: 12g
- Fat: 8g
- Carbohydrates: 50g
- Fiber: 7g

Apple Cinnamon Overnight Oats

- *Total Time:* 5 minutes (plus overnight soaking)
- *Servings:* 1

Ingredients:
- 1/2 cup rolled oats
- 1/2 cup unsweetened almond milk
- 1/2 medium apple, grated
- 1 tablespoon chia seeds
- 1/2 teaspoon ground cinnamon
- 1 tablespoon maple syrup
- Sliced almonds for topping

Directions:
1. In a jar or container, combine rolled oats, almond milk, grated apple, chia seeds, cinnamon, and maple syrup.
2. Stir well, cover, and refrigerate overnight.
3. In the morning, give the oats a good stir and top with sliced almonds before serving.

Nutritional Information (per serving):
- Calories: 350
- Protein: 8g
- Fat: 10g
- Carbohydrates: 60g
- Fiber: 10g

Breakfast Burrito with Black Beans and Salsa

- *Total Time:* 15 minutes
- *Servings:* 2

Ingredients:
- 4 whole wheat tortillas
- 4 large eggs, scrambled
- 1 cup black beans, cooked
- 1/2 cup salsa
- 1 avocado, sliced
- Fresh cilantro for garnish (optional)

Directions:
1. Warm the tortillas in a skillet or microwave.
2. Divide the scrambled eggs, black beans, and salsa among the tortillas.
3. Top with sliced avocado and garnish with fresh cilantro if desired.
4. Roll up each burrito, folding in the sides as you go.

Nutritional Information (per serving):
- Calories: 420
- Protein: 18g
- Fat: 20g
- Carbohydrates: 45g
- Fiber: 12g

Almond Butter Toast with Sliced Strawberries

- *Total Time:* 5 minutes
- *Servings:* 1

Ingredients:
- 2 slices whole grain bread, toasted
- 2 tablespoons almond butter
- 1 cup strawberries, sliced
- Drizzle of honey (optional)

Directions:
1. Spread almond butter evenly on the toasted bread slices.
2. Arrange sliced strawberries on top.
3. Drizzle with honey if desired.

Nutritional Information (per serving):
- Calories: 350
- Protein: 10g
- Fat: 18g
- Carbohydrates: 40g
- Fiber: 8g

Veggie and Cheese Frittata

- *Total Time:* 20 minutes
- *Servings:* 4

Ingredients:
- 6 large eggs
- 1/2 cup milk
- Salt and pepper to taste
- 1 tablespoon olive oil
- 1 bell pepper, diced

* 1 cup cherry tomatoes, halved
* 1 cup spinach, chopped
* 1/2 cup feta cheese, crumbled

Directions:

1. Preheat the oven to 350°F (175°C).
2. In a bowl, whisk together eggs, milk, salt, and pepper.
3. Heat olive oil in an oven-safe skillet over medium heat.
4. Add diced bell pepper and cook until softened.
5. Add cherry tomatoes and spinach, cooking until the spinach wilts.
6. Pour the egg mixture over the veggies and sprinkle with crumbled feta.
7. Transfer the skillet to the oven and bake for about 15 minutes or until the frittata is set.

Nutritional Information (per serving):

* Calories: 220
* Protein: 15g
* Fat: 15g
* Carbohydrates: 8g
* Fiber: 2g

Turmeric and Ginger Infused Smoothie

* *Total Time:* 10 minutes
* *Servings:* 1

Ingredients:

* 1 cup almond milk
* 1/2 banana, frozen
* 1/2 teaspoon ground turmeric

- 1/2 teaspoon fresh ginger, grated
- 1 tablespoon chia seeds
- 1 tablespoon honey (optional)
- Ice cubes

Directions:

1. In a blender, combine almond milk, frozen banana, turmeric, ginger, chia seeds, and honey.
2. Blend until smooth and creamy.
3. Add ice cubes and blend again until desired consistency is reached.
4. Pour into a glass and enjoy.

Nutritional Information (per serving):

- Calories: 230
- Protein: 6g
- Fat: 8g
- Carbohydrates: 35g
- Fiber: 7g

Lunch

Quinoa and Black Bean Salad

- *Total Time:* 20 minutes
- *Servings:* 4

Ingredients:
- 1 cup quinoa, cooked and cooled
- 1 can (15 oz) black beans, drained and rinsed
- 1 cup cherry tomatoes, halved
- 1 cucumber, diced
- 1/4 cup red onion, finely chopped
- 1/4 cup fresh cilantro, chopped
- 2 tablespoons olive oil
- Juice of 1 lime
- Salt and pepper to taste
- Feta cheese crumbles for garnish (optional)

Directions:
1. In a large bowl, combine cooked quinoa, black beans, cherry tomatoes, cucumber, red onion, and cilantro.
2. In a small bowl, whisk together olive oil, lime juice, salt, and pepper.
3. Pour the dressing over the quinoa mixture and toss until well combined.
4. Garnish with feta cheese crumbles if desired.

Nutritional Information (per serving):
- Calories: 320
- Protein: 12g
- Fat: 10g
- Carbohydrates: 48g
- Fiber: 10g

Grilled Chicken Caesar Wrap

- *Total Time:* 15 minutes
- *Servings:* 2

Ingredients:

- 2 whole wheat tortillas
- 1 grilled chicken breast, sliced
- 1 cup romaine lettuce, chopped
- 1/4 cup Caesar dressing
- 1/4 cup parmesan cheese, grated
- Black pepper to taste

Directions:

1. Lay out the tortillas and divide the sliced grilled chicken between them.
2. Top with chopped romaine lettuce.
3. Drizzle Caesar dressing over the lettuce and sprinkle with grated parmesan cheese.
4. Season with black pepper to taste.
5. Roll up each tortilla to create wraps.

Nutritional Information (per serving):

- Calories: 380
- Protein: 25g
- Fat: 18g
- Carbohydrates: 30g
- Fiber: 6g

Lentil and Vegetable Soup

- *Total Time:* 30 minutes
- *Servings:* 6

Ingredients:
- 1 cup dried green lentils, rinsed
- 1 onion, diced
- 2 carrots, sliced
- 2 celery stalks, chopped
- 3 cloves garlic, minced
- 6 cups vegetable broth
- 1 can (14 oz) diced tomatoes
- 1 teaspoon ground cumin
- 1 teaspoon smoked paprika
- Salt and pepper to taste
- Fresh parsley for garnish (optional)

Directions:
1. In a large pot, combine lentils, onion, carrots, celery, garlic, vegetable broth, diced tomatoes, cumin, and smoked paprika.
2. Bring to a boil, then reduce heat and simmer until lentils and vegetables are tender (about 20-25 minutes).
3. Season with salt and pepper to taste.
4. Garnish with fresh parsley if desired.

Nutritional Information (per serving):
- Calories: 220
- Protein: 14g
- Fat: 1g
- Carbohydrates: 40g
- Fiber: 15g

Greek Salad with Grilled Shrimp

- *Total Time:* 20 minutes
- *Servings:* 4

Ingredients:

- 1 pound large shrimp, peeled and deveined
- 1 tablespoon olive oil
- 1 teaspoon dried oregano
- Salt and pepper to taste
- 1 cucumber, diced
- 1 cup cherry tomatoes, halved
- 1/2 red onion, thinly sliced
- 1 cup Kalamata olives, pitted
- 1 cup feta cheese, crumbled
- 1/4 cup fresh parsley, chopped
- Greek dressing

Directions:

1. In a bowl, toss shrimp with olive oil, dried oregano, salt, and pepper.
2. Grill shrimp until opaque and cooked through.
3. In a large salad bowl, combine diced cucumber, cherry tomatoes, red onion, Kalamata olives, feta cheese, and chopped parsley.
4. Add grilled shrimp to the salad.
5. Drizzle with Greek dressing and toss gently to combine.

Nutritional Information (per serving):

- Calories: 350
- Protein: 25g
- Fat: 20g
- Carbohydrates: 15g
- Fiber: 5g

Zucchini Noodles with Pesto and Cherry Tomatoes

- *Total Time:* 15 minutes
- *Servings:* 2

Ingredients:

- 4 medium zucchinis, spiralized into noodles
- 1 cup cherry tomatoes, halved
- 1/2 cup fresh basil leaves
- 1/4 cup pine nuts
- 1/4 cup grated Parmesan cheese
- 1/3 cup olive oil
- 2 cloves garlic, minced
- Salt and pepper to taste

Directions:

1. In a food processor, combine basil, pine nuts, Parmesan cheese, olive oil, and minced garlic.
2. Blend until smooth, adding more olive oil if needed.
3. Season the pesto with salt and pepper to taste.
4. In a large pan, sauté zucchini noodles until just tender.
5. Toss zucchini noodles with pesto and cherry tomatoes until well coated.

Nutritional Information (per serving):

- Calories: 320
- Protein: 8g
- Fat: 28g
- Carbohydrates: 12g
- Fiber: 4g

Turkey and Avocado Lettuce Wraps

- *Total Time:* 15 minutes
- *Servings:* 2

Ingredients:

- 1/2 pound lean ground turkey
- 1 teaspoon olive oil
- 1 teaspoon taco seasoning
- Iceberg lettuce leaves (as wraps)
- 1 avocado, sliced
- 1 cup cherry tomatoes, halved
- 1/4 cup red onion, finely chopped
- Greek yogurt or sour cream for topping

Directions:

1. In a skillet, heat olive oil over medium heat.
2. Add ground turkey and cook until browned, stirring in taco seasoning.
3. Assemble lettuce wraps by placing a spoonful of turkey, avocado slices, cherry tomatoes, and red onion on each lettuce leaf.
4. Top with a dollop of Greek yogurt or sour cream.
5. Serve immediately.

Nutritional Information (per serving):

- Calories: 320
- Protein: 20g
- Fat: 18g
- Carbohydrates: 22g
- Fiber: 8g

Chickpea and Spinach Stuffed Bell Peppers

- *Total Time:* 30 minutes
- *Servings:* 4

Ingredients:

- 4 bell peppers, halved and seeds removed
- 1 can (15 oz) chickpeas, drained and rinsed
- 2 cups fresh spinach, chopped
- 1 cup quinoa, cooked
- 1/2 cup feta cheese, crumbled
- 1 teaspoon ground cumin
- Salt and pepper to taste
- Olive oil for drizzling

Directions:

1. Preheat the oven to 375°F (190°C).
2. In a bowl, combine chickpeas, chopped spinach, cooked quinoa, feta cheese, ground cumin, salt, and pepper.
3. Stuff each bell pepper half with the chickpea and spinach mixture.
4. Drizzle with olive oil.
5. Bake for 20-25 minutes or until peppers are tender.

Nutritional Information (per serving):

- Calories: 280
- Protein: 12g
- Fat: 8g
- Carbohydrates: 40g
- Fiber: 8g

Caprese Salad with Balsamic Glaze

- *Total Time:* 10 minutes
- *Servings:* 2

Ingredients:
- 2 large tomatoes, sliced
- 1 ball fresh mozzarella cheese, sliced
- Fresh basil leaves
- Balsamic glaze
- Salt and pepper to taste

Directions:
1. Arrange tomato and mozzarella slices on a serving plate.
2. Tuck fresh basil leaves between the tomato and mozzarella slices.
3. Drizzle with balsamic glaze.
4. Season with salt and pepper to taste.
5. Serve immediately.

Nutritional Information (per serving):
- Calories: 220
- Protein: 14g
- Fat: 16g
- Carbohydrates: 10g
- Fiber: 2g

Asian-Inspired Chicken Salad

- *Total Time:* 20 minutes
- *Servings:* 4

Ingredients:
- 2 cups shredded cooked chicken breast

- 1 cup shredded cabbage
- 1 cup shredded carrots
- 1 bell pepper, thinly sliced
- 1/4 cup sliced green onions
- 1/4 cup cilantro, chopped
- 1/4 cup peanuts, chopped
- Sesame ginger dressing

Directions:
1. In a large bowl, combine shredded chicken, cabbage, carrots, bell pepper, green onions, and cilantro.
2. Toss with sesame ginger dressing until well coated.
3. Garnish with chopped peanuts.
4. Serve chilled.

Nutritional Information (per serving):
- Calories: 280
- Protein: 25g
- Fat: 16g
- Carbohydrates: 12g
- Fiber: 4g

Sweet Potato and Kale Salad with Tahini Dressing

- *Total Time:* 25 minutes
- *Servings:* 4

Ingredients:
- 2 medium sweet potatoes, peeled and diced
- 1 bunch kale, stems removed and leaves torn
- 1/4 cup tahini
- 2 tablespoons olive oil

- 2 tablespoons lemon juice
- 1 clove garlic, minced
- Salt and pepper to taste
- Pomegranate seeds for garnish

Directions:
1. Roast sweet potatoes in the oven until tender.
2. Massage kale leaves with olive oil until softened.
3. In a large bowl, combine roasted sweet potatoes and massaged kale.
4. In a small bowl, whisk together tahini, olive oil, lemon juice, minced garlic, salt, and pepper.
5. Drizzle the tahini dressing over the salad.
6. Garnish with pomegranate seeds before serving.

Nutritional Information (per serving):
- Calories: 320
- Protein: 8g
- Fat: 18g
- Carbohydrates: 35g
- Fiber: 6g

Broccoli and Cheddar Stuffed Chicken Breast

- *Total Time:* 35 minutes
- *Servings:* 2

Ingredients:
- 2 boneless, skinless chicken breasts
- 1 cup broccoli florets, steamed and chopped
- 1/2 cup sharp cheddar cheese, shredded
- 1 teaspoon garlic powder
- Salt and pepper to taste
- Olive oil for brushing

Directions:

1. Preheat the oven to 375°F (190°C).
2. Cut a pocket into each chicken breast.
3. In a bowl, mix chopped broccoli, cheddar cheese, garlic powder, salt, and pepper.
4. Stuff each chicken breast with the broccoli and cheddar mixture.
5. Secure with toothpicks if needed.
6. Brush the chicken breasts with olive oil.
7. Bake for 25-30 minutes or until the chicken is cooked through.

Nutritional Information (per serving):

- Calories: 320
- Protein: 40g
- Fat: 15g
- Carbohydrates: 5g
- Fiber: 2g

Tuna Salad Lettuce Cups

- *Total Time:* 15 minutes
- *Servings:* 4

Ingredients:

- 2 cans (5 oz each) tuna, drained
- 1/4 cup mayonnaise
- 1 celery stalk, finely chopped
- 1/4 red onion, finely chopped
- 1 tablespoon Dijon mustard
- Salt and pepper to taste
- Butter lettuce leaves for cups

Directions:

1. In a bowl, mix tuna, mayonnaise, chopped celery, red onion, Dijon mustard, salt, and pepper.
2. Spoon the tuna salad into butter lettuce leaves to form cups.
3. Serve immediately.

Nutritional Information (per serving):

- Calories: 220
- Protein: 25g
- Fat: 10g
- Carbohydrates: 5g
- Fiber: 1g

Quinoa Bowl with Roasted Vegetables and Tofu

- *Total Time:* 40 minutes
- *Servings:* 2

Ingredients:

- 1 cup quinoa, cooked
- 1 cup broccoli florets
- 1 bell pepper, sliced
- 1 zucchini, sliced
- 1 cup extra-firm tofu, cubed
- 2 tablespoons olive oil
- 1 teaspoon smoked paprika
- Salt and pepper to taste
- Lemon wedges for serving

Directions:

1. Preheat the oven to 400°F (200°C).

2. Toss broccoli, bell pepper, and zucchini with olive oil, smoked paprika, salt, and pepper.
3. Spread the vegetables on a baking sheet and roast for 20-25 minutes.
4. In a separate pan, sauté tofu until golden brown.
5. Assemble bowls with quinoa, roasted vegetables, and sautéed tofu.
6. Serve with lemon wedges.

Nutritional Information (per serving):
- Calories: 380
- Protein: 20g
- Fat: 18g
- Carbohydrates: 40g
- Fiber: 6g

Eggplant and Tomato Stack with Mozzarella

- *Total Time:* 30 minutes
- *Servings:* 4

Ingredients:
- 1 large eggplant, sliced
- 2 large tomatoes, sliced
- 1 cup fresh mozzarella cheese, sliced
- 1/4 cup fresh basil leaves
- Balsamic glaze for drizzling
- Olive oil for brushing
- Salt and pepper to taste

Directions:
1. Preheat a grill or grill pan.
2. Brush eggplant slices with olive oil and season with salt and pepper.

3. Grill eggplant slices until tender, about 2-3 minutes per side.
4. Assemble stacks by layering grilled eggplant, tomato, mozzarella, and fresh basil.
5. Drizzle with balsamic glaze before serving.

Nutritional Information (per serving):
- Calories: 220
- Protein: 12g
- Fat: 15g
- Carbohydrates: 15g
- Fiber: 5g

Cauliflower Fried Rice
- *Total Time:* 25 minutes
- *Servings:* 4

Ingredients:
- 1 medium cauliflower, grated
- 2 tablespoons sesame oil
- 2 eggs, beaten
- 1 cup mixed vegetables (peas, carrots, corn)
- 1 cup cooked shrimp or chicken, diced
- 3 tablespoons soy sauce
- 1 teaspoon ginger, minced
- 2 cloves garlic, minced
- Green onions for garnish

Directions:
1. In a large pan, heat sesame oil over medium heat.
2. Add beaten eggs and scramble until cooked.
3. Stir in mixed vegetables, cooked shrimp or chicken, grated cauliflower, soy sauce, ginger, and garlic.
4. Cook until the cauliflower is tender.
5. Garnish with chopped green onions before serving.

Nutritional Information (per serving):

- Calories: 240
- Protein: 18g
- Fat: 12g
- Carbohydrates: 15g
- Fiber: 5g

Dinner

Baked Salmon with Lemon and Dill

- *Total Time:* 25 minutes
- *Servings:* 2

Ingredients:

- 2 salmon fillets
- 1 lemon, thinly sliced
- 2 tablespoons fresh dill, chopped
- 2 tablespoons olive oil
- Salt and pepper to taste

Directions:

1. Preheat the oven to 375°F (190°C).
2. Place salmon fillets on a baking sheet lined with parchment paper.
3. Season with salt and pepper.
4. Drizzle olive oil over the salmon and top with lemon slices and chopped dill.
5. Bake for 15-20 minutes or until the salmon flakes easily with a fork.

Nutritional Information (per serving):

- Calories: 320
- Protein: 25g
- Fat: 22g
- Carbohydrates: 2g
- Fiber: 1g

Spaghetti Squash with Tomato and Basil Sauce

- *Total Time:* 40 minutes
- *Servings:* 4

Ingredients:

- 1 large spaghetti squash, halved and seeds removed
- 2 tablespoons olive oil
- 3 cloves garlic, minced
- 1 can (28 oz) crushed tomatoes
- 1 teaspoon dried basil
- Salt and pepper to taste
- Fresh basil for garnish
- Grated Parmesan cheese for topping

Directions:

1. Preheat the oven to 375°F (190°C).
2. Place spaghetti squash halves on a baking sheet, cut side down.
3. Bake for 30-35 minutes or until the squash is tender.
4. In a pan, heat olive oil and sauté minced garlic until fragrant.
5. Add crushed tomatoes, dried basil, salt, and pepper. Simmer for 10 minutes.
6. Scrape the spaghetti squash with a fork to create "noodles."
7. Top with tomato and basil sauce, garnish with fresh basil, and sprinkle with Parmesan cheese.

Nutritional Information (per serving):

- Calories: 180
- Protein: 4g
- Fat: 8g

- Carbohydrates: 28g
- Fiber: 6g

Lemon Garlic Roasted Chicken Thighs

- *Total Time:* 40 minutes
- *Servings:* 4

Ingredients:

- 4 bone-in, skin-on chicken thighs
- 2 lemons, juiced and zested
- 4 cloves garlic, minced
- 2 tablespoons olive oil
- 1 teaspoon dried thyme
- Salt and pepper to taste
- Fresh parsley for garnish

Directions:

1. Preheat the oven to 400°F (200°C).
2. In a bowl, mix lemon juice, lemon zest, minced garlic, olive oil, dried thyme, salt, and pepper.
3. Place chicken thighs in a baking dish and pour the lemon-garlic mixture over them.
4. Roast for 30-35 minutes or until the chicken reaches an internal temperature of 165°F (74°C).
5. Garnish with fresh parsley before serving.

Nutritional Information (per serving):

- Calories: 320
- Protein: 22g
- Fat: 24g
- Carbohydrates: 6g
- Fiber: 1g

Shrimp and Asparagus Stir-Fry

- *Total Time:* 20 minutes
- *Servings:* 4

Ingredients:

- 1 pound shrimp, peeled and deveined
- 1 bunch asparagus, trimmed and cut into 2-inch pieces
- 2 tablespoons soy sauce
- 1 tablespoon hoisin sauce
- 1 tablespoon sesame oil
- 2 cloves garlic, minced
- 1 teaspoon ginger, minced
- 1 tablespoon olive oil
- Sesame seeds for garnish

Directions:

1. In a bowl, mix soy sauce, hoisin sauce, sesame oil, minced garlic, and minced ginger.
2. Heat olive oil in a wok or large pan over high heat.
3. Add shrimp and stir-fry until pink and opaque.
4. Add asparagus and continue to stir-fry until tender-crisp.
5. Pour the sauce over the shrimp and asparagus, tossing to coat evenly.
6. Garnish with sesame seeds before serving.

Nutritional Information (per serving):

- Calories: 250
- Protein: 30g
- Fat: 10g
- Carbohydrates: 10g
- Fiber: 3g

Eggplant Parmesan with Whole Wheat Pasta

- *Total Time:* 50 minutes
- *Servings:* 6

Ingredients:
- 1 large eggplant, sliced
- 2 cups whole wheat pasta, cooked
- 2 cups marinara sauce
- 1 cup mozzarella cheese, shredded
- 1/2 cup Parmesan cheese, grated
- Fresh basil for garnish

Directions:
1. Preheat the oven to 375°F (190°C).
2. Arrange eggplant slices on a baking sheet and bake for 20 minutes, flipping halfway through.
3. In a baking dish, layer cooked whole wheat pasta, marinara sauce, baked eggplant slices, and cheeses.
4. Repeat the layers, finishing with a layer of cheese on top.
5. Bake for 20-25 minutes or until the cheese is melted and bubbly.
6. Garnish with fresh basil before serving.

Nutritional Information (per serving):
- Calories: 380
- Protein: 18g
- Fat: 15g
- Carbohydrates: 45g
- Fiber: 10g

Teriyaki Turkey Lettuce Wraps

- *Total Time:* 30 minutes
- *Servings:* 4

Ingredients:
- 1 pound ground turkey
- 1/4 cup low-sodium soy sauce
- 2 tablespoons teriyaki sauce
- 1 tablespoon honey
- 1 tablespoon sesame oil
- 2 cloves garlic, minced
- 1 teaspoon ginger, grated
- Butter lettuce leaves for wrapping
- Sliced green onions and sesame seeds for garnish

Directions:
1. In a skillet, cook ground turkey over medium heat until browned.
2. In a bowl, whisk together soy sauce, teriyaki sauce, honey, sesame oil, minced garlic, and grated ginger.
3. Pour the teriyaki sauce over the cooked turkey, stirring to combine.
4. Spoon the turkey mixture onto butter lettuce leaves.
5. Garnish with sliced green onions and sesame seeds.
6. Serve immediately.

Nutritional Information (per serving):
- Calories: 280
- Protein: 22g
- Fat: 16g
- Carbohydrates: 12g
- Fiber: 2g

Butternut Squash and Sage Risotto

- *Total Time:* 45 minutes
- *Servings:* 4

Ingredients:
- 1 cup Arborio rice
- 2 cups butternut squash, diced
- 1 onion, finely chopped
- 4 cups vegetable broth, heated
- 1/2 cup dry white wine
- 2 tablespoons fresh sage, chopped
- 1/4 cup Parmesan cheese, grated
- Salt and pepper to taste

Directions:
1. In a large pan, sauté onions in olive oil until translucent.
2. Add Arborio rice and cook for 1-2 minutes.
3. Pour in white wine and stir until mostly absorbed.
4. Add diced butternut squash and chopped sage.
5. Gradually add hot vegetable broth, stirring frequently until rice is cooked and squash is tender.
6. Stir in Parmesan cheese, salt, and pepper.
7. Serve hot.

Nutritional Information (per serving):
- Calories: 320
- Protein: 8g
- Fat: 4g
- Carbohydrates: 60g
- Fiber: 5g

Cilantro Lime Grilled Chicken

- *Total Time:* 25 minutes
- *Servings:* 4

Ingredients:
- 4 boneless, skinless chicken breasts
- 1/4 cup fresh cilantro, chopped
- Zest and juice of 2 limes
- 2 tablespoons olive oil
- 2 cloves garlic, minced
- Salt and pepper to taste

Directions:
1. In a bowl, mix chopped cilantro, lime zest, lime juice, olive oil, minced garlic, salt, and pepper.
2. Marinate chicken breasts in the cilantro-lime mixture for at least 15 minutes.
3. Preheat the grill or grill pan.
4. Grill chicken for 6-7 minutes per side or until fully cooked.
5. Let the chicken rest for a few minutes before slicing.
6. Serve warm.

Nutritional Information (per serving):
- Calories: 250
- Protein: 30g
- Fat: 12g
- Carbohydrates: 2g
- Fiber: 0g

Quinoa Stuffed Bell Peppers with Black Beans

- *Total Time:* 40 minutes
- *Servings:* 4

Ingredients:

- 4 bell peppers, halved and seeds removed
- 1 cup quinoa, cooked
- 1 can (15 oz) black beans, drained and rinsed
- 1 cup corn kernels
- 1 cup salsa
- 1 teaspoon cumin
- 1/2 teaspoon chili powder
- Shredded cheddar cheese for topping
- Fresh cilantro for garnish

Directions:

1. Preheat the oven to 375°F (190°C).
2. In a bowl, mix cooked quinoa, black beans, corn, salsa, cumin, and chili powder.
3. Stuff each bell pepper half with the quinoa mixture.
4. Top with shredded cheddar cheese.
5. Bake for 25-30 minutes or until peppers are tender.
6. Garnish with fresh cilantro before serving.

Nutritional Information (per serving):

- Calories: 350
- Protein: 12g
- Fat: 8g
- Carbohydrates: 60g
- Fiber: 10g

Baked Cod with Mediterranean Salsa

- *Total Time:* 30 minutes
- *Servings:* 4

Ingredients:
- 4 cod fillets
- 1 cup cherry tomatoes, halved
- 1/2 cucumber, diced
- 1/4 cup Kalamata olives, pitted and sliced
- 1/4 cup red onion, finely chopped
- 2 tablespoons fresh parsley, chopped
- 2 tablespoons olive oil
- Juice of 1 lemon
- Salt and pepper to taste

Directions:
1. Preheat the oven to 400°F (200°C).
2. Season cod fillets with salt and pepper and place them on a baking sheet.
3. In a bowl, combine cherry tomatoes, cucumber, Kalamata olives, red onion, parsley, olive oil, and lemon juice to make the salsa.
4. Spoon the Mediterranean salsa over the cod fillets.
5. Bake for 15-20 minutes or until the cod is flaky.
6. Serve hot.

Nutritional Information (per serving):
- Calories: 280
- Protein: 30g
- Fat: 14g
- Carbohydrates: 10g
- Fiber: 3g

Stir-Fried Tofu with Broccoli and Sesame Seeds

- *Total Time:* 25 minutes
- *Servings:* 4

Ingredients:
- 1 block firm tofu, pressed and cubed
- 2 cups broccoli florets
- 2 tablespoons soy sauce
- 1 tablespoon sesame oil
- 1 tablespoon rice vinegar
- 1 tablespoon maple syrup
- 1 tablespoon cornstarch
- 2 tablespoons sesame seeds
- Green onions for garnish

Directions:
1. In a bowl, whisk together soy sauce, sesame oil, rice vinegar, maple syrup, and cornstarch.
2. In a wok or large pan, stir-fry cubed tofu until golden brown.
3. Add broccoli florets and continue stir-frying until tender-crisp.
4. Pour the sauce over tofu and broccoli, tossing to coat evenly.
5. Sprinkle sesame seeds over the stir-fry.
6. Garnish with sliced green onions.
7. Serve over rice or noodles.

Nutritional Information (per serving):
- Calories: 280
- Protein: 16g
- Fat: 18g
- Carbohydrates: 20g
- Fiber: 4g

Grilled Vegetable and Goat Cheese Quesadillas

- *Total Time:* 30 minutes
- *Servings:* 4

Ingredients:
- 8 whole wheat tortillas
- 2 zucchinis, sliced
- 1 red bell pepper, sliced
- 1 yellow bell pepper, sliced
- 1 cup goat cheese, crumbled
- Olive oil for brushing
- Fresh cilantro for garnish

Directions:
1. Preheat a grill or grill pan.
2. Brush zucchini and bell pepper slices with olive oil.
3. Grill vegetables until tender and slightly charred.
4. Lay out flour tortillas and spread goat cheese evenly over each.
5. Top with grilled vegetables and cover with remaining tortillas.
6. Grill quesadillas for 2-3 minutes per side or until cheese is melted.
7. Garnish with fresh cilantro.
8. Slice and serve.

Nutritional Information (per serving):
- Calories: 350
- Protein: 12g
- Fat: 18g
- Carbohydrates: 38g
- Fiber: 6g

Spinach and Mushroom Quiche

- *Total Time:* 50 minutes
- *Servings:* 6

Ingredients:

- 1 pie crust (store-bought or homemade)
- 1 cup fresh spinach, chopped
- 1 cup mushrooms, sliced
- 1 cup feta cheese, crumbled
- 4 large eggs
- 1 cup milk
- Salt and pepper to taste
- Fresh parsley for garnish

Directions:

1. Preheat the oven to 375°F (190°C).
2. Line a pie dish with the pie crust.
3. In a skillet, sauté spinach and mushrooms until wilted.
4. Spread the sautéed vegetables and feta cheese over the pie crust.
5. In a bowl, whisk together eggs, milk, salt, and pepper.
6. Pour the egg mixture over the vegetables and cheese.
7. Bake for 30-35 minutes or until the quiche is set and golden brown.
8. Garnish with fresh parsley.
9. Allow to cool slightly before slicing.

Nutritional Information (per serving):

- Calories: 280
- Protein: 12g
- Fat: 20g

- Carbohydrates: 15g
- Fiber: 2g

Turkey and Sweet Potato Skillet

- *Total Time:* 35 minutes
- *Servings:* 4

Ingredients:

- 1 pound ground turkey
- 2 sweet potatoes, peeled and diced
- 1 onion, finely chopped
- 2 cloves garlic, minced
- 1 teaspoon smoked paprika
- 1 teaspoon cumin
- Salt and pepper to taste
- Fresh cilantro for garnish
- Avocado slices for serving

Directions:

1. In a skillet, brown ground turkey over medium heat.
2. Add diced sweet potatoes, chopped onion, and minced garlic.
3. Season with smoked paprika, cumin, salt, and pepper.
4. Cover and simmer until sweet potatoes are tender.
5. Garnish with fresh cilantro.
6. Serve with avocado slices on the side.

Nutritional Information (per serving):

- Calories: 320
- Protein: 20g
- Fat: 15g
- Carbohydrates: 25g
- Fiber: 4g

Mediterranean Chickpea Salad

- *Total Time:* 15 minutes
- *Servings:* 4

Ingredients:

- 2 cans (15 oz each) chickpeas, drained and rinsed
- 1 cucumber, diced
- 1 cup cherry tomatoes, halved
- 1/2 red onion, finely chopped
- 1/2 cup feta cheese, crumbled
- Kalamata olives, pitted and sliced
- Fresh parsley, chopped
- Olive oil and lemon juice for dressing
- Salt and pepper to taste

Directions:

1. In a large bowl, combine chickpeas, diced cucumber, cherry tomatoes, chopped red onion, feta cheese, olives, and fresh parsley.
2. Drizzle with olive oil and lemon juice.
3. Season with salt and pepper.
4. Toss gently to combine.
5. Serve chilled.

Nutritional Information (per serving):

- Calories: 280
- Protein: 14g
- Fat: 12g
- Carbohydrates: 32g
- Fiber: 8g

Snacks

Hummus and Veggie Sticks

- *Total Time:* 10 minutes
- *Servings:* 4

Ingredients:

- 1 cup hummus
- Carrot sticks
- Cucumber slices
- Bell pepper strips
- Cherry tomatoes

Directions:

1. Arrange hummus in a serving bowl.
2. Wash and cut carrot sticks, cucumber slices, bell pepper strips, and cherry tomatoes.
3. Serve the veggie sticks with hummus for dipping.

Nutritional Information (per serving):

- Calories: 120
- Protein: 5g
- Fat: 7g
- Carbohydrates: 12g
- Fiber: 5g

Almond and Coconut Energy Bites

- *Total Time:* 15 minutes
- *Servings:* 12

Ingredients:

- 1 cup almonds, toasted
- 1 cup shredded coconut

- 1/2 cup dates, pitted
- 1 tablespoon chia seeds
- 1/4 cup almond butter
- 1 teaspoon vanilla extract
- Pinch of sea salt

Directions:
1. In a food processor, combine almonds, shredded coconut, dates, chia seeds, almond butter, vanilla extract, and sea salt.
2. Pulse until the mixture forms a sticky dough.
3. Roll the dough into bite-sized balls.
4. Refrigerate for at least 1 hour before serving.

Nutritional Information (per serving):
- Calories: 90
- Protein: 3g
- Fat: 6g
- Carbohydrates: 8g
- Fiber: 2g

Edamame with Sea Salt
- *Total Time:* 5 minutes
- *Servings:* 2

Ingredients:
- 2 cups edamame, steamed
- Sea salt to taste

Directions:
1. Steam edamame according to package instructions.
2. Sprinkle it with sea salt.
3. Toss to coat evenly.
4. Serve in a bowl for a simple and nutritious snack.

Nutritional Information (per serving):

- Calories: 180
- Protein: 16g
- Fat: 8g
- Carbohydrates: 15g
- Fiber: 8g

Greek Yogurt with Honey and Walnuts

- *Total Time:* 5 minutes
- *Servings:* 2

Ingredients:

- 2 cups Greek yogurt
- 2 tablespoons honey
- 1/4 cup walnuts, chopped

Directions:

1. Spoon Greek yogurt into serving bowls.
2. Drizzle honey over the yogurt.
3. Sprinkle chopped walnuts on top.
4. Serve for a protein-packed and satisfying snack.

Nutritional Information (per serving):

- Calories: 300
- Protein: 20g
- Fat: 15g
- Carbohydrates: 25g
- Fiber: 2g

Apple Slices with Almond Butter

- *Total Time:* 5 minutes
- *Servings:* 2

Ingredients:
- 2 apples, sliced
- 4 tablespoons almond butter

Directions:
1. Slice apples into wedges.
2. Spread almond butter on each apple slice.
3. Arrange on a plate and enjoy this quick and nutritious snack.

Nutritional Information (per serving):
- Calories: 220
- Protein: 5g
- Fat: 15g
- Carbohydrates: 20g
- Fiber: 5g

Hard-Boiled Eggs with Paprika

- *Total Time:* 15 minutes
- *Servings:* 4

Ingredients:
- 4 large eggs
- Paprika for sprinkling
- Salt and pepper to taste

Directions:
1. Place eggs in a saucepan and cover with water.
2. Bring water to a boil, then reduce heat and simmer for 10 minutes.

3. Remove eggs from water and let them cool.
4. Peel eggs and sprinkle with paprika, salt, and pepper.
5. Enjoy this protein-packed snack.

Nutritional Information (per serving):
- Calories: 70
- Protein: 6g
- Fat: 5g
- Carbohydrates: 0g
- Fiber: 0g

Cottage Cheese with Pineapple Chunks

- *Total Time:* 5 minutes
- *Servings:* 2

Ingredients:
- 1 cup cottage cheese
- 1/2 cup pineapple chunks, fresh or canned

Directions:
1. Spoon cottage cheese into serving bowls.
2. Top with pineapple chunks.
3. Mix gently and enjoy this sweet and savory snack.

Nutritional Information (per serving):
- Calories: 200
- Protein: 15g
- Fat: 8g
- Carbohydrates: 15g
- Fiber: 1g

Mixed Nuts and Dried Fruit Trail Mix

- *Total Time:* 5 minutes
- *Servings:* 4

Ingredients:

- 1 cup mixed nuts (almonds, walnuts, cashews)
- 1/2 cup dried fruit (raisins, cranberries, apricots)

Directions:

1. Combine mixed nuts and dried fruit in a bowl.
2. Toss to mix evenly.
3. Portion into snack-sized servings.
4. Enjoy this energy-boosting trail mix.

Nutritional Information (per serving):

- Calories: 250
- Protein: 6g
- Fat: 18g
- Carbohydrates: 20g
- Fiber: 3g

Avocado and Tomato Salsa

- *Total Time:* 10 minutes
- *Servings:* 2

Ingredients:

- 1 ripe avocado, diced
- 1 cup cherry tomatoes, halved
- 1/4 red onion, finely chopped
- 1/4 cup fresh cilantro, chopped
- Lime juice for drizzling
- Salt and pepper to taste

Directions:
1. In a bowl, combine diced avocado, cherry tomatoes, red onion, and cilantro.
2. Drizzle with lime juice and season with salt and pepper.
3. Mix gently and enjoy with whole-grain crackers or vegetable sticks.

Nutritional Information (per serving):
- Calories: 200
- Protein: 3g
- Fat: 15g
- Carbohydrates: 15g
- Fiber: 7g

Roasted Chickpeas with Cumin and Paprika

- *Total Time:* 40 minutes
- *Servings:* 4

Ingredients:
- 2 cans (15 oz each) chickpeas, drained and rinsed
- 2 tablespoons olive oil
- 1 teaspoon ground cumin
- 1 teaspoon paprika
- Salt and pepper to taste

Directions:
1. Preheat the oven to 400°F (200°C).
2. Pat chickpeas dry with a paper towel.
3. In a bowl, toss chickpeas with olive oil, cumin, paprika, salt, and pepper.
4. Spread chickpeas on a baking sheet in a single layer.

5. Roast for 30-35 minutes or until chickpeas are crispy.
6. Let them cool before serving.

Nutritional Information (per serving):
- Calories: 220
- Protein: 9g
- Fat: 8g
- Carbohydrates: 29g
- Fiber: 8g

Dessert

Chocolate Avocado Mousse

- *Total Time:* 15 minutes
- *Servings:* 4

Ingredients:
- 2 ripe avocados
- 1/2 cup dark cocoa powder
- 1/4 cup maple syrup
- 1 teaspoon vanilla extract
- A pinch of salt
- Fresh berries for garnish (optional)

Directions:
1. Scoop avocados into a blender or food processor.
2. Add cocoa powder, maple syrup, vanilla extract, and a pinch of salt.
3. Blend until smooth and creamy.
4. Divide into serving bowls and refrigerate for at least 1 hour.
5. Garnish with fresh berries before serving.

Nutritional Information (per serving):
- Calories: 200
- Protein: 3g
- Fat: 15g
- Carbohydrates: 20g
- Fiber: 8g

Coconut Flour Banana Bread

- *Total Time:* 1 hour
- *Servings:* 8

Ingredients:

- 3 ripe bananas, mashed
- 3 eggs
- 1/4 cup coconut oil, melted
- 1 teaspoon vanilla extract
- 1/2 cup coconut flour
- 1 teaspoon baking soda
- A pinch of salt
- 1/2 cup chopped walnuts (optional)

Directions:

1. Preheat the oven to 350°F (180°C). Grease a loaf pan.
2. In a bowl, mix mashed bananas, eggs, melted coconut oil, and vanilla extract.
3. Add coconut flour, baking soda, and salt. Mix until well combined.
4. Fold in chopped walnuts if desired.
5. Pour the batter into the prepared loaf pan.
6. Bake for 45-50 minutes or until a toothpick comes out clean.
7. Allow to cool before slicing.

Nutritional Information (per serving):

- Calories: 180
- Protein: 4g
- Fat: 12g
- Carbohydrates: 18g
- Fiber: 4g

Chia Seed Pudding with Mango

- *Total Time:* 4 hours (includes chilling time)
- *Servings:* 2

Ingredients:
- 1/4 cup chia seeds
- 1 cup almond milk
- 1 tablespoon maple syrup
- 1/2 teaspoon vanilla extract
- 1 ripe mango, diced

Directions:
1. In a bowl, whisk together chia seeds, almond milk, maple syrup, and vanilla extract.
2. Let it sit for 15 minutes, then whisk again to prevent clumping.
3. Cover and refrigerate for at least 4 hours or overnight.
4. Before serving, layer chia pudding with diced mango.
5. Enjoy this refreshing and nutritious dessert.

Nutritional Information (per serving):
- Calories: 220
- Protein: 6g
- Fat: 9g
- Carbohydrates: 32g
- Fiber: 11g

Baked Apples with Cinnamon and Walnuts

- *Total Time:* 40 minutes
- *Servings:* 4

Ingredients:

- 4 apples, cored and halved
- 1/4 cup chopped walnuts
- 2 tablespoons maple syrup
- 1 teaspoon ground cinnamon
- 1/4 cup water

Directions:

1. Preheat the oven to 375°F (190°C).
2. Place apple halves in a baking dish.
3. In a bowl, mix chopped walnuts, maple syrup, and ground cinnamon.
4. Spoon the mixture into the center of each apple half.
5. Pour water into the baking dish.
6. Cover with foil and bake for 20 minutes. Remove foil and bake for an additional 15-20 minutes or until the apples are tender.
7. Serve warm.

Nutritional Information (per serving):

- Calories: 180
- Protein: 2g
- Fat: 5g
- Carbohydrates: 35g
- Fiber: 6g

Raspberry Almond Bliss Balls

- *Total Time:* 20 minutes
- *Servings:* 12

Ingredients:

- 1 cup almonds
- 1 cup dried raspberries
- 1/4 cup shredded coconut
- 2 tablespoons almond butter
- 1 tablespoon maple syrup
- 1/2 teaspoon almond extract

Directions:

1. In a food processor, pulse almonds until finely ground.
2. Add dried raspberries, shredded coconut, almond butter, maple syrup, and almond extract.
3. Process until the mixture comes together.
4. Roll into bite-sized balls.
5. Refrigerate for at least 1 hour before serving.

Nutritional Information (per serving):

- Calories: 90
- Protein: 3g
- Fat: 6g
- Carbohydrates: 8g
- Fiber: 3g

Greek Yogurt Popsicles with Berries

- *Total Time:* 6 hours (includes freezing time)
- *Servings:* 6

Ingredients:

- 2 cups Greek yogurt
- 1 cup mixed berries (strawberries, blueberries, raspberries)
- 2 tablespoons honey
- 1 teaspoon vanilla extract

Directions:

1. In a bowl, mix Greek yogurt, honey, and vanilla extract until well combined.
2. Gently fold in mixed berries.
3. Spoon the mixture into popsicle molds.
4. Insert popsicle sticks and freeze for at least 6 hours or overnight.
5. Run molds under warm water to release popsicles.
6. Enjoy these refreshing and protein-packed treats!

Nutritional Information (per serving):

- Calories: 120
- Protein: 8g
- Fat: 2g
- Carbohydrates: 18g
- Fiber: 2g

Pumpkin Pie Smoothie Bowl

- *Total Time:* 10 minutes
- *Servings:* 2

Ingredients:

- 1 cup pumpkin puree
- 1 frozen banana
- 1/2 cup Greek yogurt
- 1/2 cup almond milk
- 1 teaspoon pumpkin spice
- 2 tablespoons maple syrup
- Granola and chopped nuts for topping

Directions:

1. In a blender, combine pumpkin puree, frozen banana, Greek yogurt, almond milk, pumpkin spice, and maple syrup.
2. Blend until smooth and creamy.
3. Pour into bowls and top with granola and chopped nuts.
4. Serve immediately and savor the flavors of fall.

Nutritional Information (per serving):

- Calories: 220
- Protein: 6g
- Fat: 4g
- Carbohydrates: 45g
- Fiber: 6g

Chocolate Covered Strawberries

- *Total Time:* 20 minutes
- *Servings:* 4

Ingredients:

- 1 pint fresh strawberries, washed and dried
- 1/2 cup dark chocolate chips
- 1 tablespoon coconut oil
- Chopped nuts or shredded coconut for garnish (optional)

Directions:

1. In a microwave-safe bowl, melt dark chocolate chips and coconut oil in 30-second intervals, stirring until smooth.
2. Dip each strawberry into the melted chocolate, coating evenly.
3. Place on a parchment-lined tray.
4. Optional: Sprinkle chopped nuts or shredded coconut on top.
5. Refrigerate for 10-15 minutes or until chocolate hardens.
6. Indulge in these delightful and simple chocolate-covered strawberries.

Nutritional Information (per serving):

- Calories: 120
- Protein: 2g
- Fat: 8g
- Carbohydrates: 15g
- Fiber: 4g

Almond Joy Chia Seed Pudding

- *Total Time:* 4 hours (includes chilling time)
- *Servings:* 2

Ingredients:

- 1/4 cup chia seeds
- 1 cup almond milk
- 2 tablespoons shredded coconut
- 2 tablespoons chocolate chips
- 2 tablespoons sliced almonds
- 1 tablespoon maple syrup

Directions:

1. In a bowl, whisk together chia seeds, almond milk, shredded coconut, chocolate chips, sliced almonds, and maple syrup.
2. Let it sit for 15 minutes, then whisk again to prevent clumping.
3. Cover and refrigerate for at least 4 hours or overnight.
4. Stir before serving and enjoy this delicious and nutritious pudding.

Nutritional Information (per serving):

- Calories: 250
- Protein: 5g
- Fat: 18g
- Carbohydrates: 20g
- Fiber: 10g

Pistachio and Cranberry Bark

- *Total Time:* 1 hour (includes chilling time)
- *Servings:* 8

Ingredients:
- 1 cup dark chocolate, melted
- 1/2 cup pistachios, shelled and chopped
- 1/4 cup dried cranberries

Directions:
1. Line a baking sheet with parchment paper.
2. Pour melted dark chocolate onto the parchment paper, spreading it evenly.
3. Sprinkle chopped pistachios and dried cranberries over the melted chocolate.
4. Refrigerate for at least 30 minutes or until the bark hardens.
5. Break into pieces and enjoy this sweet and crunchy treat.

Nutritional Information (per serving):
- Calories: 150
- Protein: 2g
- Fat: 10g
- Carbohydrates: 15g
- Fiber: 3g

Smoothies

Green Goddess Smoothie with Spinach and

- *Total Time:* 5 minutes
- *Servings:* 2

Ingredients:
- 2 cups fresh spinach
- 1 cup pineapple chunks (fresh or frozen)
- 1 banana, peeled
- 1/2 avocado, peeled and pitted
- 1 cup coconut water
- Ice cubes (optional)

Directions:
1. In a blender, combine fresh spinach, pineapple chunks, banana, avocado, and coconut water.
2. Blend until smooth and creamy.
3. Add ice cubes if a colder consistency is desired.
4. Pour into glasses and enjoy this nutrient-packed green goddess smoothie.

Nutritional Information (per serving):
- Calories: 180
- Protein: 3g
- Fat: 7g
- Carbohydrates: 30g
- Fiber: 8g

Berry Blast Smoothie with Greek Yogurt

- *Total Time:* 5 minutes
- *Servings:* 2

Ingredients:

- 1 cup mixed berries (strawberries, blueberries, raspberries)
- 1/2 cup Greek yogurt
- 1 banana, peeled
- 1 tablespoon honey
- 1 cup almond milk
- Ice cubes (optional)

Directions:

1. In a blender, combine mixed berries, Greek yogurt, banana, honey, and almond milk.
2. Blend until smooth and creamy.
3. Add ice cubes if desired for a colder texture.
4. Pour into glasses and savor the delightful flavors of this berry blast smoothie.

Nutritional Information (per serving):

- Calories: 180
- Protein: 8g
- Fat: 3g
- Carbohydrates: 35g
- Fiber: 6g

Mango Turmeric Smoothie

- *Total Time:* 5 minutes
- *Servings:* 2

Ingredients:
- 1 cup mango chunks (fresh or frozen)
- 1 banana, peeled
- 1/2 teaspoon ground turmeric
- 1 tablespoon chia seeds
- 1 cup coconut milk
- Ice cubes (optional)

Directions:
1. In a blender, combine mango chunks, banana, ground turmeric, chia seeds, and coconut milk.
2. Blend until smooth and vibrant.
3. Add ice cubes for a refreshing touch if desired.
4. Pour into glasses and enjoy the tropical goodness of this mango turmeric smoothie.

Nutritional Information (per serving):
- Calories: 220
- Protein: 4g
- Fat: 10g
- Carbohydrates: 30g
- Fiber: 6g

Peanut Butter Banana Protein Smoothie

- *Total Time:* 5 minutes
- *Servings:* 2

Ingredients:
- 2 ripe bananas, peeled
- 2 tablespoons peanut butter
- 1 scoop vanilla protein powder
- 1 cup almond milk
- 1/2 teaspoon cinnamon
- Ice cubes (optional)

Directions:
1. In a blender, combine ripe bananas, peanut butter, vanilla protein powder, almond milk, and cinnamon.
2. Blend until smooth and creamy.
3. Add ice cubes if a colder consistency is preferred.
4. Pour into glasses and relish the rich and protein-packed goodness of this peanut butter banana smoothie.

Nutritional Information (per serving):
- Calories: 280
- Protein: 15g
- Fat: 12g
- Carbohydrates: 35g
- Fiber: 5g

Tropical Paradise Smoothie with Coconut Water

- *Total Time:* 5 minutes
- *Servings:* 2

Ingredients:

- 1 cup pineapple chunks (fresh or frozen)
- 1/2 cup mango chunks (fresh or frozen)
- 1/2 cup papaya chunks (fresh or frozen)
- 1/2 cup coconut water
- 1 tablespoon lime juice
- Ice cubes (optional)

Directions:

1. In a blender, combine pineapple chunks, mango chunks, papaya chunks, coconut water, and lime juice.
2. Blend until smooth and refreshing.
3. Add ice cubes if desired for an extra chill.
4. Pour into glasses and transport yourself to a tropical paradise with this delightful smoothie.

Nutritional Information (per serving):

- Calories: 160
- Protein: 2g
- Fat: 1g
- Carbohydrates: 40g
- Fiber: 5g

Kale and Pineapple Detox Smoothie

- *Total Time:* 5 minutes
- *Servings:* 2

Ingredients:

- 2 cups kale, stems removed
- 1 cup pineapple chunks (fresh or frozen)
- 1 green apple, cored and chopped
- 1/2 cucumber, peeled and sliced
- 1 tablespoon fresh ginger, grated
- 1 cup coconut water
- Ice cubes (optional)

Directions:

1. In a blender, combine kale, pineapple chunks, green apple, cucumber, fresh ginger, and coconut water.
2. Blend until smooth and detoxifying.
3. Add ice cubes if a colder texture is desired.
4. Pour into glasses and enjoy the refreshing and nutrient-packed goodness of this detox smoothie.

Nutritional Information (per serving):

- Calories: 150
- Protein: 4g
- Fat: 1g
- Carbohydrates: 36g
- Fiber: 6g

Blueberry Almond Butter Smoothie

- *Total Time:* 5 minutes
- *Servings:* 2

Ingredients:
- 1 cup blueberries (fresh or frozen)
- 2 tablespoons almond butter
- 1 banana, peeled
- 1 cup almond milk
- 1 tablespoon honey
- Ice cubes (optional)

Directions:
1. In a blender, combine blueberries, almond butter, banana, almond milk, and honey.
2. Blend until smooth and creamy.
3. Add ice cubes for a colder consistency.
4. Pour into glasses and savor the delightful combination of blueberries and almond butter in this smoothie.

Nutritional Information (per serving):
- Calories: 250
- Protein: 6g
- Fat: 14g
- Carbohydrates: 30g
- Fiber: 5g

Coffee and Almond Milk Smoothie

- *Total Time:* 5 minutes
- *Servings:* 2

Ingredients:

- 1 cup brewed coffee, cooled
- 1 banana, peeled
- 1/2 cup Greek yogurt
- 1 cup almond milk
- 1 tablespoon almond butter
- 1 teaspoon honey
- Ice cubes (optional)

Directions:

1. In a blender, combine brewed coffee, banana, Greek yogurt, almond milk, almond butter, and honey.
2. Blend until smooth and energizing.
3. Add ice cubes for a refreshing touch.
4. Pour into glasses and relish the fusion of coffee and almond flavors in this invigorating smoothie.

Nutritional Information (per serving):

- Calories: 180
- Protein: 8g
- Fat: 8g
- Carbohydrates: 24g
- Fiber: 4g

Cucumber Mint Green Smoothie

- *Total Time:* 5 minutes
- *Servings:* 2

Ingredients:
- 2 cups spinach
- 1 cucumber, peeled and sliced
- 1/2 cup mint leaves
- 1 green apple, cored and chopped
- 1/2 lemon, juiced
- 1 cup water
- Ice cubes (optional)

Directions:
1. In a blender, combine spinach, cucumber, mint leaves, green apple, lemon juice, and water.
2. Blend until smooth and refreshing.
3. Add ice cubes for an extra chill.
4. Pour into glasses and enjoy the crispness of this cucumber mint green smoothie.

Nutritional Information (per serving):
- Calories: 80
- Protein: 2g
- Fat: 1g
- Carbohydrates: 20g
- Fiber: 5g

Strawberry Kiwi Smoothie with Chia Seeds

- *Total Time:* 5 minutes
- *Servings:* 2

Ingredients:
- 1 cup strawberries, hulled
- 2 kiwis, peeled and sliced
- 1 banana, peeled
- 1 tablespoon chia seeds
- 1 cup coconut water
- Ice cubes (optional)

Directions:
1. In a blender, combine strawberries, kiwis, banana, chia seeds, and coconut water.
2. Blend until smooth and full of tropical flavors.
3. Add ice cubes for a cooler experience.
4. Pour into glasses and relish the sweetness of this strawberry kiwi smoothie with chia seeds.

Nutritional Information (per serving):
- Calories: 150
- Protein: 3g
- Fat: 2g
- Carbohydrates: 35g
- Fiber: 8g

Conclusion

In reaching the conclusion of this transformative journey towards health and wellness for women over 50 through the realm of intermittent fasting, it is essential to reflect on the profound impact such dietary choices can have on one's overall well-being. The culmination of the recipes, insights, and guidance within this cookbook is not merely an endpoint but the beginning of a sustained, healthier lifestyle.

As you close the pages of this cookbook, consider it not as the end but the initiation of a new chapter in your life—one where nourishing your body becomes an art, and intermittent fasting serves as the brushstroke that shapes this masterpiece. The recipes provided are not mere concoctions; they are gateways to a vibrant and energetic life, tailored to the unique needs of women navigating the golden years.

The diverse array of recipes presented here is a celebration of nutritional diversity. From nutrient-rich breakfasts to satisfying dinners, each dish contributes to the mosaic of essential vitamins, minerals, and macronutrients necessary for sustaining vitality. The intentional inclusion of a variety of ingredients ensures not only a flavorful culinary experience but also a well-rounded nutritional profile that addresses the changing requirements of the body over 50.

Central to this journey is the practice of intermittent fasting—a scientifically backed approach that extends beyond a mere dietary trend. The strategic intervals of fasting and feasting create a metabolic dance that enhances cellular function, supports weight management, and potentially contributes to increased longevity. More than a diet plan, intermittent fasting becomes a lifestyle shift, fostering mindful eating habits and a harmonious relationship with food.

Acknowledging that each woman's journey is unique, it's essential to recognize that challenges may arise. Whether adapting to new eating patterns, experimenting with unfamiliar ingredients, or fine-tuning the balance of fasting windows, challenges are opportunities for growth. Embrace them as stepping stones rather than stumbling blocks, knowing that every effort contributes to the profound tapestry of your wellness journey.

True wellness is sustainable, rooted in habits that withstand the tests of time. As you integrate the principles of intermittent fasting into your daily life, remember that patience and consistency are your allies. Small, positive changes compound over time, leading to lasting improvements in energy levels, mental clarity, and overall health.

This cookbook is more than a collection of recipes; it's a reminder of the importance of self-care. Nourishing your body with wholesome, thoughtfully prepared meals is an act of self-love. Take the time to savor the flavors, appreciate the journey of crafting each dish, and revel in the joy that comes with prioritizing your health.

As you embark on this journey, take a moment to express gratitude for your body, which has carried you through the years with resilience and strength. Extend this gratitude to those who have contributed to your well-being—the farmers who cultivate the ingredients, the chefs who inspired these recipes, and the supportive community that surrounds you.

Your journey to health and wellness is not finite; it's an ongoing odyssey. Continue to explore, adapt, and evolve as you discover what works best for your body. Embrace the dynamic nature of this expedition, recognizing that wellness is not a destination but a continuous process of self-discovery and growth.

In concluding this cookbook, envision it not as a manual with a final chapter but as a guide that propels you towards sustained health, vitality, and joy. May the recipes within these pages be a source of inspiration, the intermittent fasting principles a compass, and the experience an enduring testament to your commitment to a healthier, more vibrant you. As you close this chapter, know that your journey is just beginning—a journey towards a life of wellness, mindful nourishment, and the boundless potential that comes with embracing the wisdom and strength that each passing year brings.